Bipolar Disorder

Understanding Bipolar Disorder, and how it can be managed, treated, and improved

Table of Contents

Introduction 1

Chapter 1: What Is Bipolar Disorder? 2

Chapter 2: Signs & Symptoms of Bipolar Disorder 10

Chapter 3: How to Improve Bipolar Disorder Naturally or Alternatively 16

Chapter 4: Common Treatments for Bipolar Disorder 26

Chapter 5: How to Help Others with Bipolar Disorder 34

Chapter 6: Consequences of Lack of Treatment 39

Conclusion 42

Introduction

Thank you for taking the time to read this book on Bipolar Disorder!

This book covers the topic of Bipolar Disorder and will discuss in detail what exactly Bipolar Disorder is, the different ways it may present itself, what causes it in the first place, and how it can be managed and treated. You will also be presented with a list of ways you can help a loved one who is currently suffering from Bipolar Disorder.

At the completion of this book you will have a good understanding of Bipolar Disorder, and what you can do to improve and manage it. It can be a difficult condition to live with, both for the sufferer, and for those around them. Fortunately, there are strategies and treatments available that can greatly improve the symptoms associated with Bipolar Disorder, particularly if it is diagnosed quickly.

Please keep in mind that this book does not aim to serve as medical advice, but rather as an overall guide to Bipolar Disorder and our current knowledge of it. Before self-diagnosing or undergoing any treatment methods, always consult a medical professional.

Once again, thanks for choosing this book, I hope you find it to be helpful!

Chapter 1: What Is Bipolar Disorder?

Mental Health, according to Merriam and Webster, is the state of being sound rationally and candidly, in mind and in cognitive processes. In addition, this also means that a person is healthy, with no psychological sickness or disorder. This could also mean that the individual feels good about themselves, has positive sentiments about others, and has the confident capacity to face the challenges life throws at them.

Emotional wellness directly influences everything we do, including our social, physical, and spiritual capacity. It is vital to be healthy mentally because it helps us to make the correct decisions, even under extreme pressure, and helps us get to know other people socially. Our holistic psychological well-being is imperative to our formation at each stage of life.

Over the span of a person's life, they may develop a mental health disorder. There are several factors that can contribute to this development, which we have listed below:

Biological Factors: when we say biological factors, this includes microorganisms, cell societies, human endoparasites, and parts from microorganisms that can harm the overall wellbeing of a person. This can determine a person's capacity to either be immune to diseases or to be susceptible to them.

Life Experiences: Mental challenges may occur when an individual has experienced trauma, abuse, or pain. When a person encounters a horrible event, say abuse or an accident, several symptoms can present themselves. This may be right away, or further down the line, such as with PTSD.

Hereditary or Genetic: Scientists believe that psychological disorders or mental illnesses are also caused by an assortment of hereditary and human ecological elements. Usually, when a person has a blood relative that has been diagnosed with any type of mental illness, they have a higher chance of developing one too.

After we experience something horrifying, our mind and body can respond in an unexpected way. Our minds were designed to put up a wall to shield us from remembering and going through the same pain again. Even though our innate response can be attributed to a primal reaction, the way we react to certain occasions is generally because of how our brains work. Nonetheless, for individuals who have not gone through anything traumatizing that may trigger a mental relapse or disorder, it is still remarkably important to have our psychological well-being in check.

According to research conducted by the National Institute for Mental Health in 2015, the United States alone experienced a 33% increase in the number of individuals affected with mental illness. In fact, America spends $193.2 billion each year treating mental illness, with suicide being the 10th leading cause of death.

Statistics show that:

• Roughly 1 in 5 adults in the U.S. experiences psychological instability

• Roughly 1 in every 25 adults in the U.S. experiences a period of genuine psychological instability each year

• Around 1 out of 5 youth in the 13-18-year-old age group encounters an extreme mental turmoil in this age period

- 1.1% of adults in the U.S. live with schizophrenia, a chronic and severe mental illness that majorly affects how a person is in touch with reality

- 2.6% of adults in the U.S. live with bipolar disorder

- 6.9% of adults in the U.S. had at least one major depressive episode in the last year

- 18.1% of adults in the U.S. have experienced anxiety, posttraumatic episodes, and/or obsessive-compulsive disorders in their lifetime

- Among the 20.2 million adults in the U.S. who have experienced substance abuse, 50.05% are affected by mental illness

- At least 26% of destitute adults remaining in asylums live with genuine psychological disorders, and an expected 46% live with serious dysfunctional behavior and substance abuse

- Roughly 20% of state detainees and 21% of nearby correctional facility detainees have "an ongoing history" of a psychological condition wherein they are thrust into rehabilitation care

- 70% of the individuals in the adolescent age group who have experienced at least one mental disorder, have gone through a deeply traumatizing event, and no less than 20% of them are still living with a mental disorder

- In the past year, 41% of adults in the U.S. living with a mental disorder received treatment. Among these patients, only 62.9% are being given continuous mental care and support

- More than 50% of mental disorders among individuals start on or before the age of 14, and more than three quarters the incidences by the time they reach the age of 25

Under the broad term of 'mental illness', there are numerous types of disorders, with the most common being: Anxiety and Panic Disorders, Schizophrenia, Bipolar Disorder, Substance Abuse & Addiction, Depression, and Eating Disorders.

The objective of this book is to lay out in full detail one of America's most common mental illness; Bipolar Disorder. This book will carefully elaborate upon what it means to be in a sensitive mental state, and what to do if you know someone who is currently dealing with Bipolar Disorder.

According to the National Institute of Mental Health, Bipolar Disorder affects approximately 5.7 million Americans – roughly around 2.6% of the U.S. population each year. Even though mental disorders can appear later in life, the average age a person develops bipolar disorder in America is at 25 years old.

This illness does not discriminate by race, age, ethnic group, social class, or gender. In fact, the number of men and women with this illness is almost equal. According to additional research, it is also possible that Bipolar Disorder is hereditary, since more than 70% of the people with this disorder have at least one relative who has experienced it themselves.

Bipolar Disorder is a kind of mental illness that causes bizarre changes in disposition, vitality, action levels, and the capacity to perform everyday tasks. There are four fundamental types of bipolar issues, and every one of them involves clear changes in the state of mind, enthusiasm, and movement levels of the person affected. When an individual experiences extreme shifts in mood – from ecstatic to depressed in the bat of an eye, they could be experiencing Bipolar Disorder. Most of the time, Bipolar Disorder is accompanied by episodes of depression, and when this happens, they last for an average of two weeks. On the other hand, a Bipolar Disorder episode alone can last anywhere from a few days up to weeks, or even months in some cases.

Currently, there is no known cure for Bipolar Disorder, however, there are numerous treatments, including therapy, that can help to manage and control the manic episodes.

There are four types of Bipolar Disorders: Bipolar Disorder I, Bipolar Disorder II, Cyclothymic Disorder, and other specified bipolar-related disorders. The first two are the most common types of Bipolar Disorder, and the fundamental contrast between Bipolar Disorder I and Bipolar Disorder II lies in the seriousness of the episodes caused by each type. For example, with Bipolar Disorder I, the manic episodes are more extreme than with Bipolar Disorder II, whilst the latter causes something many refer to as hypomania, or, in other words, a less serious type of manic behavior.

A mania, or what mental health specialists also refer to as a "manic episode", is a depressive state where the individual has a hard time finding a settled and sensible state of mind. Individuals who are in a hyper stage are extremely restless, make unreasonable choices, and commonly risk their lives by engaging in dangerous activities.

Bipolar Disorder I

To be diagnosed with Bipolar Disorder I, an individual must have experienced at least one manic episode and one major clinically depressive episode. Some call this type of bipolar disorder "classic" or often times "text-book bipolar disorder" as it is the most common. An individual may show insane indications, for example, dreams of greatness, or grand hallucinations.

Bipolar Disorder I can cause hyper-manic stages, which are severe when compared to Bipolar Disorder II. Manic episodes of Bipolar Disorder I may be so extreme that they can require hospital care. Characterizations of manic episodes include, but are not limited to the following:

- Sleep deprivation
- Peculiar high energy
- Dangerous behaviors (The need to participate in dangerous behaviors)
- Anxiety
- Having trouble concentrating
- Euphoria
- Racing thoughts

The key contrast between Bipolar Disorder I and Bipolar Disorder II is the omnipresence of mania, versus hypomania. It is vital to comprehend this distinction in detail. The mania experienced with Bipolar Disorder I is usually much more extreme and dangerous than that shown in Bipolar Disorder II.

Amidst a depressive state, an individual may feel depleted, blameworthy for reasons unknown, useless, and bad-tempered. He or she will lose interest in exercising, and therefore, may encounter sudden weight loss or gain. Suicidal thoughts can also occur in some more extreme cases.

These depressive periods can last for a considerable length of time and are often mistaken for chronic depression. An episode can't be formally considered hyper if it's caused by external factors such as alcohol, drugs, or other health conditions that may be related to having a mental illness.

Bipolar Disorder II

Bipolar Disorder II is a type of psychological instability that is similar to Bipolar Disorder I, wherein states of mind cycle between high and low. Nonetheless, in Bipolar Disorder II, the mania or episodes are never as extreme as Bipolar Disorder I.

The less-extraordinary heightened states of mind in Bipolar Disorder II are called hypomanic scenes, or hypomania.

A hypomanic episode is a period of time wherein the symptoms are less extreme; however, the individual's conduct varies from the ordinary. The distinctions may be obvious to friends and family who spend a lot of time around the person afflicted.

A hypomanic scene isn't viewed as hypomania if it's affected by medications, or any form of substance, including alcohol.

The indications of hypomania are similar to mania - a heightened state of mind, increased confidence, and an energetic disposition. Aside from that, they don't essentially affect a person's daily activities too extremely.

Cyclothymia or Cyclothymic Disorder

This type of Bipolar Disorder is generally mellow and mild. In Cyclothymia, temperaments swing between brief periods of gentle depression, and hypomania. Cyclothymic episodes never achieve the seriousness of real depressive or full lunacy episodes. Individuals with cyclothymic disorder have milder symptoms compared to the first two types of Bipolar Disorders.

In Cyclothymia, states of mind change from gentle despondency to hypomania and back. In most individuals, the example is sporadic and capricious. These periods of hypomania and depression can each keep going for a considerable length of time, respectively. Between these mood swings, some individuals may experience ordinary mind-sets for several months. On the other hand, some will cycle ceaselessly from hypomanic to discouraged, with no typical period in the middle.

When the manic episodes become severe, or depression becomes elevated, an individual no longer has Cyclothymia; rather, the individual now has Bipolar Disorder. The development of these more serious symptoms can occur at any time, and this is when most individuals will initially seek treatment.

There are no proven medications that cure Cyclothymia, but there are options to help manage the episodes, including stabilizers like lithium or lamotrigine. Antidepressants such as Prozac, Zoloft, or Paxil are often prescribed, but only for those who have experienced a full manic episode, which, by definition, does not happen in Cyclothymia. Antidepressants alone do not cure manic episodes, which are trademark qualities of Cyclothymia.

Cyclothymia may wreak havoc on the individuals who experience this mental illness. The symptoms can put a strain on an individual's capacity to perform in the workplace, along with causing relationship problems. Individuals who experience Cyclothymic episodes are also more likely to mishandle medications, and abuse alcohol. In fact, approximately 50% of Cyclothymic patients are alcohol dependent, or have abused alcohol in the past.

If Cyclothymic symptoms remain present for an extended period of time, the likelihood that people will develop Bipolar I or Bipolar II is increased. Experts feel that stabilizers may reduce the risk of this transition, but there is still a lot of research to be done to determine the best course of treatment for Cyclothymia.

Chapter 2: Signs & Symptoms of Bipolar Disorder

Signs versus Symptoms

First, let us differentiate these two words from each other so that we can have a better understanding of Bipolar Disorder, and how it presents itself.

A sign is something you can see. As a friend, a relative, or someone close to the person who is experiencing a depressive state, there are several signs that can pose as official triggers. It is extremely important you pay close attention to potential signs, as they will serve as a warning that Bipolar Disorder may be present.

A symptom, on the other hand, is something that can be felt. If you feel like you are extremely sad, or otherwise, out of the ordinary, this is a symptom. A symptom may not be obvious to the outside world, and that's why it's important to seek help as soon as you feel out of the ordinary.

If you know someone who seems to show signs and symptoms of Bipolar Disorder (or any other mental disorder), talk with them and if possible, take them to a mental health specialist. A psychiatrist can talk to them and perform certain tests to examine and analyze their state. From then, they will be able to determine whether the individual has Bipolar Disorder, or any other type of mental disorder. Their findings will incorporate an audit of both the individual's therapeutic history, and any side effects they have experienced which could be related to mental health.

When going in for a consultation, it is best to bring a companion – a relative or someone close to the individual. They might have the capacity to answer inquiries regarding the individual's conduct that the individual will be unable to answer precisely. If the individual feels that they may be bipolar, it's important that they let the mental health specialist know. Sometimes, a blood test may be performed. However, there are no direct indications of mental illness like Bipolar Disorder that can be seen in the blood. Blood tests may however, be able to check other conceivable reasons for an individual's conduct or behavior, such as hormonal imbalances.

There is a difference between depression and Bipolar Disorder (though they have many similarities). With Bipolar Disorder, an individual will experience both periods of depression, as well as periods of mania. Here is a list of the different ways that both depression and mania may present themselves:

Mania	Depression
Feeling Excessively Upbeat	Feeling Dismal or Sad For Significant Periods of Time
Having A Diminished Requirement for Rest	Pulling Back from Loved Ones
Talking Quickly	Losing Enthusiasm for Exercise
Feeling Fretful or Imprudent	Having A Huge Change in Cravings
Easily Distracted	Feeling Serious Weakness, or Absence of Enthusiasm
Trouble Focusing on One Task	Having Issues with Memory, Fixation, And Basic Leadership
Taking Part in Dangerous Activities	Suicidal Thoughts

In general, during the onset of any type of mental illnesses, the symptoms may be hard to see, most especially in individuals with Bipolar Disorder. Since this type of mental illness involves extreme mood swings which can take places over several months, it often takes a while to diagnose accurately.

The following are several symptoms that are common to a person suffering from mental illness:

Sleep and Rest Complications

Individuals who have Bipolar Disorder often have rest and sleep complications. Sometimes, they are extremely restless and may use a week's worth of energy in just a day. And yet, even if they go through a hyper stage, they may not rest and never feel tired at all. In fact, even with only a few hours of rest every night, they may still be completely energetic.

In some cases, it is the opposite where they always feel tired and constantly want to sleep. Amid a depressive stage, they may rest excessively and feel tired constantly, which is common to those who are in a depressive state. They constantly feel like they are being sucked in by a black hole of sadness, giving up all hope and wanting to sleep all their worries away instead. This sign present in depression, which is why many Bipolar Disorder patients are mistaken to be "just depressed".

Mental health specialists suggest following a customary rest plan. This is one of the initial steps they prescribe for bipolar patients to ensure that the individuals have a balanced sleep and awake routine to keep the episodes in check.

Peculiarly High Energy

Bipolar Disorder is often described as extreme scenes of insanity and misery, because when people are experiencing an episode, they are out of their normal state of mind. In any case, hypomania, or, in other words, a manifestation of the disorder, is a high-vitality state in which an individual feels overwhelming energy, however, hasn't lost his or her hold on the real world.

In fact, some mental health specialists consider hypomania to be a fascinating state because an individual's state of mind can be raised, they have a lot of vitality and imagination, and they may encounter happiness. This is the "up" side of bipolar disorder that a few people with the condition should appreciate—while it endures.

Love for Dangerous Behaviors

When they are in a hyper stage, individuals with Bipolar Disorder can have an excessive amount of confidence, which makes them feel high and mighty – like they can do anything in the world. They feel vainglorious and don't think about outcomes; everything sounds great to them and they are prone to engaging in risky behaviors.

Two of the most widely recognized risky behaviors seen in patients with Bipolar Disorder are abnormal sexual conduct, also known as paraphilia, and excessive spending.

Anxiety and Depression

An individual who is in a bipolar depressive state looks like somebody who is depressed. Similar to the symptoms of being just plain "sad", they will exhibit symptoms related to vitality, cravings, and rest.

Ordinary antidepressants alone don't usually function well in patients who are bipolar. They can even make individuals cycle between states quicker, compounding their condition. An incorrect prescription or therapy can worsen their condition, so it's always best to bring them to a mental health specialist for careful and precise evaluation of their mental health.

Having Trouble Concentrating

Having a house with tasks halfway done is another sign of Bipolar Disorder.

People who constantly jump from errand to errand and are easily distracted by the thoughts in their mind will have a feeling of wanting to start new tasks repeatedly. They will leave things undone and hop to the next task without thought.

Don't get it wrong though – some people who are mentally healthy also take on several tasks and never get to finish any of them. We're talking about numerous tasks – up to hundreds of different tasks in a day without finishing any of them.

Work-Related Challenges

Individuals with Bipolar Disorder regularly experience issues at work. The symptoms associated with Bipolar Disorder can meddle with their capacity to appear for work, carry out their tasks, and connect beneficially with others.

Notwithstanding having issues finishing tasks and concentrating, they may also experience issues resting, peevishness, the presence of an inflated self-image amid a hyper stage, and depression during other stages. A considerable measure of the working environment issues are due to difficulties in maintaining relationships.

Alcohol or Substance Abuse

More than half of the people diagnosed with Bipolar Disorder also have a history of substance or alcohol abuse. Most patients will drink when they are in a hyper stage to set them at a slower pace, and on the opposite, drink when they feel discouraged, in hopes of bringing their temperament up.

Racing Thoughts

Racing thoughts is a side effect that might be difficult to detect because it happens inside the mind of a person and isn't visually obvious. However, it can contribute to a person entering into panic mode. Individuals who experience racing thoughts feel like their brain is going a hundred miles an hour and they can't control or slow down their thoughts. This can be an overwhelming and scary thing to experience.

Overly Talkative

Of course, there are some people without any mental health issues that could be considered talkative. However, an individual who is overly talkative is a standout. Amongst the most widely recognized indications of Bipolar Disorder, being overly talkative and even talking to themselves is a common sign. The individual will talk quickly to themselves as if having an actual conversation with another person. It is also common for them to talk over the top of others without listening or paying proper attention to the conversation at hand.

Chapter 3: How to Improve Bipolar Disorder Naturally or Alternatively

Normally, mental health specialists treat Bipolar Disorder with a blend of prescribed medicines and psychotherapy. Temper stabilizers are often the primary medications utilized in treatments and may be needed to be taken for some time. Lithium has been a broadly utilized drug of choice and is often the go-to stabilizer. However, it has a few potential side effects like impacting the thyroid, joint torment, and heartburn in some patients.

Another option is the use of Antipsychotics, especially during periods of hyper-activity. The mental health specialist may begin with a low dosage of the medication to check how an individual reacts and may gradually increase it over time. In the long run, a patient may be given a blend of medications to control their symptoms.

Keep in mind that all medications may have potential side effects. In case a patient is pregnant or is taking other medications, it is extremely important to let the mental health specialist know before they prescribe any pharmaceuticals.

Some mental health specialists recommend keeping a diary or any form of a written journal that can help during treatment. The journal will help monitor states of mind, eating and resting patterns, and may become a written reminder to the patient of the special occasions and milestones they have experienced. In addition, this journal will serve as a guide to the mental health specialist to know whether the current treatment is working. If the symptoms do not regress, the mental health specialist may arrange certain adjustments in the medicines or an alternate kind of psychotherapy.

There is no known cure for Bipolar Disorder. However, with the appropriate treatment and support from family and friends, the patient can absolutely manage the episodes of the disorder.

It also helps if friends and family close to the patient learn as much as they can about Bipolar Disorder. In addition, it's also useful for the patient to know about and understand Bipolar Disorder and how it manifests. Knowing why you're experiencing certain symptoms and having some idea of what to expect, can help to keep people more level-headed when dealing with mental health issues.

A greater understanding of Bipolar Disorder has the potential of repairing stressed relationships. Close relatives and friends may also help during the treatment of Bipolar Disorder, and being aware of the symptoms and treatments may help them be more understanding when the patient acts out or experiences mood swings.

A number of individuals diagnosed with Bipolar Disorder have revealed that choosing alternative medicines or natural ways to treat the said disorder helped them minimize the side effects of prescriptions drugs. As stated before, there is no known cure for Bipolar Disorder, and much more study needs to be done. The efficacy of alternative medicines has not been fully tested, but anecdotally, there are certainly some positive results.

Alternative medicines are not replacements for actual pharmaceuticals. In fact, many patients believe that blending alternative and prescription medicines has advantages. Bipolar Disorder requires overseeing two unmistakable classes of side effects, including hyperactivity manifestations that may induce unreasonable mood swings, nervousness, and anxiety, while the depressive side effects may include eating disorders, and a lack of zest in life. Any treatment can potentially cause a swing too far in either direction, and so it's vitally important that symptoms are monitored closely when any new treatment is started.

Complementary and Alternative Medicine (CAM) has corresponding solutions for many types of mental illness. Several people who have been diagnosed with Bipolar Disorder invest a large part of their daily energy to these types of treatments, which the National Institute of Health supports.

In any case, the use of CAM treatments should not encourage a patient to discard their antidepressants. If for example, a mental health specialist should require the patient to take stimulants, they should still take these accordingly, and not self-prescribe.

There are several ways to treat Bipolar Disorder with medications, but for those who prefer to do it naturally or with alternative medicine, there are a couple of options. This chapter will discuss some of the alternative options for treating Bipolar Disorder.

Natural Treatments and Therapy

Proper Diet – The right food and eating plan is important, especially for those diagnosed with Bipolar Disorder. A recent study showed that 68% of Bipolar Disorder patients were overweight or obese. Additionally, individuals with diabetes, low bone density, or cardiovascular disease are more at risk of developing Bipolar Disorder.

A well-prepared food plan can lessen the danger of these conditions, or even eliminate them entirely.

Normal dietary patterns for Bipolar Disorder should help patients retain their strength and prevent them from putting on additional weight. Although Bipolar Disorder is a mental health issue, having a proper diet plan actually affects how the mind functions. Medications that may be given alongside a proper diet include Serotonin, Noradrenaline, and Dopamine.

Serotonin is a chemical neurotransmitter in the human body that has a correlation to feelings of happiness. When a person produces enough serotonin, it can affect their mood, appetite, digestion, memory, social, and sexual behavior. Additionally, when serotonin levels are low, the person may have intense desires for sugary sweets like chocolates and ice cream.

Medical health specialists advise patients to "science their pushcart" by making a list of the things they need at the supermarket prior to the trip. This way, it's easier for individuals stick to their diet plan and maintain a healthy, well-balanced diet throughout the treatment.

Adequate Rest – Consistent, well-balanced rest is imperative for individuals with Bipolar Disorder. Being diagnosed with a mental illness can mess up an individual's overall sleeping routine. Sometimes, patients want to sleep the whole day and they will still feel tired, but sometimes it is the exact opposite, wherein rest appears to be unnecessary. Not getting enough rest and sleep can trigger a change in an individual's state of mind, making them restless, anxious, and compulsive. Getting enough rest, on the other hand, is essential in making sure the individual feels light, well-rested, and energetic.

In order to get quality rest, a person may need to set a schedule, and make changes to their sleeping environment. Individuals must make sure that the room is dark and comfortable. It's recommended that they also stay away from any form of electronic screens (TV, smartphones, tablets, laptop or computers) before heading to bed. Avoiding eating a heavy meal or consuming alcohol before bed is also important.

Adequate Exercise - Moderate and consistent exercise can affect a person's state of mind and can help fend off many illnesses such as cardiovascular diseases, bone diseases, and diabetes. There is not enough medical evidence to definitively prove that exercise can assist individuals with Bipolar Disorder, however informal studies and anecdotal evidence suggests that it might provide some benefits.

A research study conducted in 2015 recommends that any exercise or physical movement of the body may be beneficial in managing the depressive episodes of Bipolar Disorder.

More studies on the effects of exercise are expected in the coming years to help discover exactly how much exercise an individual ought to engage in, how regularly, and how exceptional the movement should be in order to achieve the greatest outcome possible.

Reflection and Meditation – individuals diagnosed with Bipolar Disorder who reflect through carefully-planned therapy sessions may see a decrease in depressive episodes that specifically correspond to how they ponder and think. The more they contemplate, the fewer episodes they typically have – especially if the contemplation was focused on positive thinking.

Care Groups and Support Groups – when an individual is going through a depressive state in their life, it is often because they feel like they are alone. Being part of a care group or support group is one of the many ways an individual can combat this loneliness. It can also be a chance for close relatives and friends to show their love and support for the patient. Finding out about others' battles and triumphs may also help the individual to overcome any difficulties they may have personally.

In the modern world, care and support groups are no longer limited to those situated in your hometown. Though is it preferable to have a face-to-face care and support group, if time and distance do not permit, there are online sites and communities that can provide support.

The Depression and Bipolar Support Alliance (DBSA) is an online group that keeps track of the success stories of members and posts them online. In addition, they also have a list of the contact data for care and support groups all over the United States, as well as detailed information about the condition, medicines, and materials that may be useful for the patient, their friends, and family.

Likewise, The National Alliance on Mental Illness (NAMI) also provides information about care and support groups across the country. They provide a great deal of useful information about Bipolar Disorder as well as other conditions.

Interpersonal and Social Rhythm Therapy (IPSRT) – is a therapy that shows individuals diagnosed with Bipolar Disorder how to keep up a normal timetable in all parts of their life, including an exercise regime, a sleep schedule, and a balanced and nutritional diet plan.

Initially created as a one-on-one type of psychotherapy, the program has since been adjusted to work in various types of settings, including inpatient and outpatient setups. IPSRT is an adjunctive treatment for individuals with focus issues, and it includes different methods to help enhance prescription adherence, and assist people during difficult times in their lives.

IPSRT is a transitory sort of treatment that empowers patients to better manage changes in social or work environments, and issues relating to other people. It helps people to deal with expressing emotions and maintaining healthy relationships.

Eye Movement Desensitization and Reprocessing Therapy (EMDR) – According to a research study performed in 2014, EMDR can help manage Bipolar Disorder episodes by using a combination of specific eye movements and the recollection of traumatic events.

Light Therapy – patients who are clinically diagnosed with Bipolar Disorder may have hindered circadian rhythms, which may imply that their daily body functions are not running correctly. However, there are procedures that may correct the natural body clock and help manage their bipolar episodes. This therapy involves changing the amount of natural light, and the amount of darkness a person is subject to during the day. This aims to reset the circadian rhythm, and help to establish a healthy sleeping pattern in patients.

Cognitive Behavioral Therapy (CBT) – Research studies demonstrate that CBT can assist patients in managing their Bipolar Disorder episodes. In 2017, a research study suggested that CBT was able to diminish the backslide rate of Bipolar Disorder and decrease depressive indications which may include insanity and psychosocial thoughts. Also, CBT was shown to help individuals with identifying negative thought patterns or practices, and help them replace these with more positive and empowering ones.

CBT empowers people to recognize and change personal conduct standards that are unsafe or ineffectual, and then replace them with simplified activities and practical approaches. CBT can help a person focus on their current issues and face them without getting stressed, depressed, or overwhelmed.

CBT can be useful for treating different aspects of mental disorders including sadness, nervousness, and anxiety.

Conventional Chinese Medicine – when people think of alternative medicine, Chinese medicine is usually one of the methods that comes to mind. Like other countries in Asia, China has a fair share of their traditional medicinal processes that they have been practicing for centuries. The Chinese methodology focuses on certain homegrown blends, extensive changes in eating routines, and everyday practices. There is currently not enough scientific evidence to either support or discount Chinese natural medicine, but there are many anecdotal reports that speak in favor of it.

Many mental health specialists are fine with their patients engaging in Chinese medicinal practices, so long as they also continue to adhere to their traditional treatments also.

Traditional Chinese healing practices may include acupuncture, traditional body massage, and tai chi, among others.

Natural Food, Vitamins, and Herbs

Rhodiola Rosea – is a long-lasting, blossoming plant that grows naturally in Europe, Asia, and North America. The roots of this plant are often used as traditional medicine for additional strength, energy, endurance, and mental health development. A research study conducted in 2017 indicates that while Rhodiola does not clinically cure depression, it can elicit fewer reactions or side effects to traditional medications when taken in conjunction with them.

It is believed that Rhodiola is a powerful adaptogen that helps the body adapt to stress. In Russia, this herb has been used for centuries to treat anxiety, fatigue, and depression.

St John's Wort – also known as Perforate St John's Wort, this is a flowering plant widely used as a medicinal herb to treat depression. It has been said that this plant has antidepressant properties, but there is minimal clinical evidence to back up these claims. In some countries, this herb is also used to treat wounds, skin irritations, and psoriasis. This healthy herb is widely believed to treat mental illnesses like anxiety and even obsessive-compulsive disorder (OCD), and may be taken as a liquid, a pill, or in tea form.

S-Adenosyl methionine, or SAMe – a coenzyme found naturally in the human body, SAMe has undergone extensive studies since it appears to have properties that help decrease the symptoms of depression, premenstrual syndrome (PMS), and even osteoarthritis. Used in alternative medicine, the use of SAMe is associated with the development, actuation, or breakdown of different synthetic compounds in the body, including phospholipids, proteins, hormones, and certain medications. Several clinical preliminaries are currently in progress to decide the most ideal approach for utilizing SAMe in individuals with mental disorders, especially Bipolar Disorder.

Omega-3 Fatty Acids – individuals diagnosed with Bipolar Disorder are recommended to eat more fish, since they are overwhelmingly fortified with Omega-3 Fatty Acids. Examples of these are mackerel, sardines, and salmon. Omega-3 is also available in nuts and plant oils.

In research studies, scientists have found that the countries that eat more fish have a lower rate of mental illnesses in comparison to those who don't eat as much. Omega-3 is known to have properties that have a calming effect on an individual.

A dose of 300 milligrams of Omega-3s is recommended to be taken every day.

Magnesium - A few clinical researchers think magnesium has certain properties that are great in managing energy levels, while managing both hyper and depressive episodes. Thus, some specialists may prescribe magnesium supplements to patients with Bipolar Disorder. Magnesium is best taken before bed, and has also been shown to assist in improving sleep quality.

Vitamins – according to testimonies, there are several people who say that vitamins play a big role in curbing Bipolar Disorder, particularly Vitamin C and Folic Acid. Analysts have discovered enough evidence that vitamin C may help, however there is currently little evidence to support the effects of folic acid on Bipolar Disorder.

Chapter 4: Common Treatments for Bipolar Disorder

Like with any other illness, physical or mental, a health specialist may prescribe medication to a patient. Common medications used for Bipolar Disorders are carbamazepine, lamotrigine, lithium, and valproic acid. These are typically coupled with observation and monitoring of the patient, just in case the prescribed medications need to be modified.

Patients diagnosed with mental disorders may experience psychosis, which is a severe mental disorder symptom that can involve hallucinations. A specialist may prescribe hospitalization if a patient is encountering chronic bouts of psychosis, or if they pose a risk to themselves or others.

If an individual encounters psychosis while taking prescription medications, they may likewise be advised to take antipsychotic medications like Quetiapine, Aripiprazole, Ziprasidone, Lurasidone, Asenapine, Olanzapine, and Risperidone.

Mental health specialists don't usually recommend antidepressants alone for an individual diagnosed with Bipolar Disorder, as they can potentially trigger manic episodes.

A mental health therapist who works with a patient diagnosed with Bipolar Disorder should regularly control the patient's treatment. Now and again, the therapist might involve other specialists, including a social worker, an advisor, and nutritionist to help create the best therapy plan for the patient.

Antipsychotic Drugs and their Side Effects

Antipsychotics, otherwise called neuroleptics are a form of sedative, which are fundamentally used to control psychosis, especially in mental illnesses like Bipolar Disorder and Schizophrenia.

Antipsychotic prescriptions are utilized as a transient treatment for Bipolar Disorder to control delusions of different kinds, hallucinations, or mania side effects. Usually, antipsychotics are taken along with calming medications, and can diminish manifestations of lunacy. These can typically be used for the long run, especially by individuals who don't respond positively to lithium and anticonvulsants.

Antipsychotic drugs help to manage the functions of the brain circuitry, particularly those that control consideration, disposition, and observation. It isn't clear how these medications function, yet they typically enhance hyper-activity.

A Mental health specialist will pay close attention to the side effects of these drugs and treatments in case there is a need to modify or take away something that may be potentially dangerous to the patient's health.

Like any medication, there are potential side effects. Although the side effects will differ from person-to-person, we have listed below the potential side effects that may be experienced as a result of using antipsychotics:

- Cardiovascular Issues Including Hypertension, And Stroke
- Gastrointestinal Issues
- Blood Issues or Problems
- Skin Conditions
- Metabolic Issues
- Sensory System Issues
- Weight Gain
- Circulatory Changes Such as an Increase or Decrease in Heart Rate

- Muscle Fatigue
- Swelling
- Diabetes
- Liver Issues
- Trouble Sleeping
- Irregular Conduct
- Seizures or Spasms
- Sexual Issues Because Of Hormonal Imbalances
- Fatigue
- Mental Trips or Episodes
- Neuroleptic Malignant Syndrome
- Suicidal Thoughts
- Hostility
- Insanity
- Pneumonia
- Dry Mouth
- Obscured Vision

While these prescription medications can provide some great benefits, they can also potentially cause the serious side effects listed above.

Below is a list of some more potential side effects, detailing what to expect if you experience them, and what medications are most likely to cause each of them:

Sexual Dysfunction – Most patients, in fact up to 43%, who take antipsychotic drugs experience some sort of sexual dysfunction. Both men and women experience this kind of side effect, especially when antipsychotic drugs are taken over the long term. This can affect everything from excitement, arousal, moxie, and even climax. According to experts, medicines like Risperidone are more likely to cause sexual dysfunction in patients compared to those who take Aripiprazole or Olanzapine.

Agranulocytosis - In uncommon cases, Clozapine may be associated with Neutropenia Agranulocytosis. This may happen to a very small portion of the patient population, quite often when first beginning treatment. This acute condition affects a person's white blood cell count and lowers it to a very dangerous level. With no white blood cells in the body, a person may have no shield against infections and diseases.

Cardiovascular Arrhythmias - All antipsychotics can add to the threat of ventricular diffusion, which can prompt a sudden heart attack. Doctors aim to abstain from using antipsychotic pharmaceuticals together with different medications that drag out the amended QT interim.

Prior to starting antipsychotic medication, the dangers and advantages should be precisely gauged, presented, and explained to patients.

Seizures - All types of antipsychotics can increase the risk of seizures.

Seizures happen when there is an abnormal and sudden mechanical activity in the brain. A person who experiences seizures could describe the sensation as similar to electric shocks in the brain which are often painful and uncontrollable, followed by body jerks and movements that are beyond a person's restraint. Epilepsy is also of the same nature, where the electrical impulses in a person's brain go beyond the normal threshold and invite a storm of electrical activity.

Metabolic Syndrome Issues – Hormonal imbalance, including weight gain, is a common side effect of using antipsychotics over the long term. An individual who experiences this may also notice a rise in blood sugar, blood pressure, and excess body fat, especially in the waist and hip area. They may also experience irregular cholesterol levels that may have a direct impact on heart diseases.

In general, the most common issues with taking antipsychotics over the long term are related to cardiovascular diseases. The older types of antipsychotics have this tendency. The newer, second-age antipsychotics, particularly Clozapine and Olanzapine, tend to cause more issues related to metabolic disorders, such as weight gain or loss, and Diabetes Mellitus.

Mental health specialists usually enroll individuals with extreme psychological disorders in close monitoring sessions, coupled with a yearly physical wellness check where heart function is examined.

The best thing to do is for an individual to let the mental health specialist know whether they have had cardiovascular issues in the past.

It is best to keep in mind that not all antipsychotics will carry these side effects. Newer medications are becoming increasingly less likely to cause adverse reactions, though you still need to be aware of the potential risks before taking any new medication.

Psychotherapy and its Side Effects

Psychotherapy, or what some call "Talk Therapy", is a treatment that aims to help people with a wide variety of dysfunctional behaviors and mental disorders.

Psychotherapy helps individuals adapt to everyday life, and better manage trauma.

There are a few distinct kinds of psychotherapy, and some will be best suited to specific conditions. Psychotherapy may also be used in conjunction with traditional pharmaceutical medicines.

Treatment might be directed in an individual, family, couple, or group setting, with most sessions lasting from 30 to 50 minutes in length. Both patient and specialist should be effectively engaged in the psychotherapy session. The trust and connection between an individual and their mental health specialist are paramount in ensuring successful psychotherapy treatment.

Psychotherapy can work rapidly to help in managing quick issues, or alternatively, be a continual and gradual process when managing longstanding and complex issues. The objectives of the treatment and the courses of action to be taken, including the frequency of the sessions, will all be dependent upon the severity of the issues at hand.

It is important that the patient still gets the right nourishment, has enough exercise and rest, and monitors their medications effectively in conjunction with the psychotherapy treatment.

Research demonstrates that most individuals who undergo psychotherapy treatments improve their mental health, and in the long run, have a higher chance of going back to their "normal life".

Around 75% of patients who enter psychotherapy demonstrate at least some form of recovery. The advantages of psychotherapy treatments include fewer manic episodes, less therapeutic issues, and increased work satisfaction.

To ensure that the patient will benefit from psychotherapy, they must cooperate with the therapist, be transparent, and should be committed to their treatment plan.

Specialists and other emotional wellness experts may propose different types of psychotherapy treatment. The type of treatment chosen will depend upon the patient's specific ailment, and the severity of their symptoms. Mental health specialists may also combine different components from multiple psychotherapy methods for the best results.

Here are some of the most common forms of psychotherapy used for treating Bipolar Disorder:

1. **Animals or Pets Therapy** – this kind of therapy uses dogs, cats, or other animals to bring solace to the patients and improve their mental, social, and emotional wellbeing. Puppies and kittens are often used in retirement homes to help the residents who are struggling with different mental disorders like Alzheimer's and Dementia. This form of therapy has also been proven to help lower blood pressure, release endorphins, provide comfort, reduce loneliness, and reduce anxiety.

2. **Behavioral Therapy** – This type of treatment tries to distinguish and help change possibly pointless or undesirable behavior patterns. It works under the assumption that all habits can be corrected and changed.

3. **Cognitive Therapy** – When Cognitive Therapy is used for mental disorders like depression and Bipolar Disorder, this treatment gives the patient a psychological toolbox that can be utilized to combat against negative thoughts.

4. **Interpersonal Therapy (IPT)** – Interpersonal is defined as relationships external to an individual – their social circle. Therefore, IPT is a type of psychotherapy that focuses on the individuals and their relationships with others.

5. **Social Rhythm Therapy (SRT)** – creates a day to day activity list for an individual, with the end goal of encouraging a healthy circadian rhythm. This is a therapy widely used to treat Bipolar Disorder.

Chapter 5: How to Help Others with Bipolar Disorder

Patients diagnosed with Bipolar Disorder might seem helpless during their emotional episodes, but they are not weak. With the right prescription medication, treatment, and daily routines, these individuals will be able to manage their episodes and in turn, go back to their lives before their disorder.

Furthermore, Bipolar Disorder can become a lot easier to deal with if friends and relatives come in and help. There are many ways to show your love and support to those who are going through this ordeal. Below is a list of the ways you can help a loved one who is currently struggling with Bipolar Disorder:

1. Teach yourself. The expression "bipolar" is tossed around a considerable measure nowadays, yet it remains broadly misunderstood. Spend some time learning more about this mental illness, and it will become easier for you to comprehend what your friend or relative is experiencing. Reading this book is a fantastic place to begin! There are also great sources like care and support groups that are available to provide more information. You may also want to check the websites of these organizations: National Institute of Mental Health, the Depression and Bipolar Support Alliance, and the International Bipolar Foundation.

2. Be understanding when they are experiencing manic episode, a mania, or a hyper stage. They may not be your ideal type of person when they're in these states, but do not hate them for it. Individuals who are diagnosed with Bipolar Disorder are managing emotional episodes that render them excessively delicate, occupied, imprudent,

and inclined to unstable behaviors – which can all be taken as a personal attack if the other person does not know about bipolar behavior. Try to be understanding, and don't take their behavior as a personal insult.

3. Channel your sympathy yet let go of the pity. The patient does not need your pity. What they need is an acknowledgment that life holds challenges for them, and that you'll be there to help them through these challenges. Just be there and sympathize with them, and with what they are going through.

4. Acknowledge that they will have good days and bad days. Whenever hyper, the individual with Bipolar Disorder can appear to be the life of the party, however, when their mood swings the other way, they may feel useless, unworthy or even hopeless. Don't add to the severity of these mood swings by getting angry with them. Instead, tell them no matter what happens, you are going to love them and that you will help them get through their ordeal.

    It is understandable that it can be difficult to know how to respond when your friend is going through an outrageous hyper or depressive period. Sometimes, it can be confusing whether you should quiet down or perk up. A great initiative is to ask how you can help, or, propose a few things that you two may do together.

5. Tune in. Listen carefully and let them know you're there to listen and to understand. Ask how they are getting along, and really tune in. In the case they talk about hurting themselves, or suicide, take it seriously and

make certain their mental health specialist is aware as soon as possible.

6. Understand that they didn't choose this illness themselves. Your friend doesn't have Bipolar Disorder because they wanted it - it is neither a character defect nor a shortcoming. Rather, investigate signs, symptoms, and sources including hereditary qualities and lifestyle factors that may be contributing to their behavior.

7. Be that friend who cares for them and looks out for them. Encouraging them to eat well, get enough exercise, get proper rest, and maintain a strategic distance from liquor and medication can really help! It does not mean you have to be their babysitter or caretaker, but having someone to check in and hold them accountable can be extremely helpful to a person suffering from Bipolar Disorder.

8. Try not to get irate if your companion quits taking their medication. They might be experiencing upsetting symptoms from prescription medication or therapy, such as weight increase or sexual dysfunction, pushing them to stop taking the medication. The best thing to do in these kinds of situations is to let them know you understand, and make sure that they visit their healthcare professional for re-evaluation.

9. Try not to abandon them. Continue showing up, continue being there, just like how you were there during their pre-bipolar days. Your friend or relative may not have the capacity to give you a warm welcome when they

see you, yet remember that it's not because they don't love you, it's simply a result of their symptoms.

10. Remain associated. People are often at a loss as to how to react when their friend is diagnosed with a mental illness. Unfortunately, the usual reaction to the diagnosis is fear, which is a big mistake. You should not let the social stigma dictate how you behave and how you treat your friend.

People who are battling mental disorders often feel disconnected and deserted. There is a big impact made by anything you can do to remain associated, regardless of how straightforward – drop by, send a note, visit just to check in, embrace them, tell them you're there if they need someone to talk to.

When somebody with Bipolar Disorder has manifestations of hypomania or insanity, occasionally they don't understand that they are acting peculiarly. A few people actually appreciate the sentiment of madness and don't want it to stop. Sometimes, when left untreated, individuals with Bipolar Disorder end up committing suicide because they feel so lost, lonely, and confused. Those who have been diagnosed are not completely safe either. Patients may discard, abuse, or simply stop taking their medications.

This can make it hard for families and close friends, who are directly impacted by the results of the medication. It can cause disputes between the individual and their family. For the most part, an adult has the privilege to decline treatment. However, they can be treated without their consent if they are found to be a danger to themselves and others.

There are also some things that individuals with Bipolar Disorder may not want you to know. At times, they may appear like they have everything under control, but as friends and family, we must remember that it could be an act. Depressed people don't always look depressed – in fact, they can appear to be perfectly fine on the outside, when that's simply not the case.

Chapter 6: Consequences of Lack of Treatment

Bipolar Disorder is a genuine psychological issue that affects around 2.3-million Americans each year. The primary reason numerous individuals with Bipolar Disorder are not being treated is that it can be difficult to diagnose, and the signs are not always easy to see.

In fact, even after analysis, treatment might be troublesome. Some people who have been analyzed and examined still stop their treatment since they feel that the prescription medication symptoms are excessively troubling, or dangerous to their body.

All of this means that many individuals with Bipolar Disorder are not getting the treatment they need.

Bipolar Disorder is a genuine psychological wellness issue that frequently goes undiscovered, misdiagnosed, and untreated.

Listed below are some of the major consequences when mental health illnesses like Bipolar Disorder are left untreated:

• Depression, dysthymic disorder, and bipolar disorder are third-ranked amongst the most common reasons for hospitalization in America, especially in individuals ages 18 to 44

• Patients who have serious mental illnesses have a heightened risk of getting chronic diseases. Americans living with serious mental illnesses die on average 25 years earlier in comparison to those who don't.

• An increasing number of America's youth aged 14 to 21 are dropping out of school due to mental health conditions.

- America has seen an increase in suicide rates. It is in fact, the 10th leading cause of death in the US and includes youth aged 10 to 14

- An average of 18 to 22 veterans commit suicide every day due to mental health issues

- Approximately 70% of individuals with Bipolar Disorder are misdiagnosed at least once before the condition is properly identified

- Up to 60% of individuals with Bipolar Disorder misuse medications or liquor

- Bipolar Disorder is the 6th leading reason for incapacity on the planet. This can result in joblessness, and relationship issues

- Postponed treatment may add to the likelihood of individuals with Bipolar Disorder abusing medications and liquor. Studies demonstrate that more than 56% of the individuals diagnosed with Bipolar Disorder are medication and alcohol abusers

- Approximately 30% of individuals with untreated Bipolar Disorder commit suicide

- Bipolar Disorder might be mistaken for some other mental and conduct issue, and the wrong treatment plan could worsen symptoms

- Untreated Bipolar Disorder can prompt social and financial issues

- Early analysis and early treatment increases the chances of improved mental health over the long term

Overall, mental health diseases affect a person's way of life – be that physically, emotionally, or spiritually. It is not something that is voluntary that an individual chooses to experience, rather, it can be caused by certain experiences in life including post-traumatic stress, abuse, hormonal imbalance, and even genetics. Mental health disorders do not choose a race, religion, political stand, color, gender, or even social status. Anyone can be affected, so it is important to take care of your holistic well-being, as well as keep an eye on the wellbeing of those around you.

Likewise, we should not feel threatened, scared, or make fun of people who have a mental disorder. If they would have it their way, they wouldn't choose to be in that predicament either.

Many people take care of their physical bodies with diet and exercise, but they oftentimes forget to take care of their mental health as well. May we always remember to take care of our psychological heath, as our minds are the control center of our whole body.

Conclusion

Thanks again for taking the time to read this book!

You should now have a good understanding of Bipolar Disorder, the treatment options available, and how to help a loved one who is suffering from Bipolar Disorder!

If you enjoyed this book, please take the time to leave me a review on Amazon. I appreciate your honest feedback, and it really helps me to continue producing high quality books.

www.ingramcontent.com/pod-product-compliance
Lightning Source LLC
LaVergne TN
LVHW020446080526
838202LV00055B/5353